Minor Illness in the Under Fives

A guide for Health Visitors

Dr. Gina Johnson
National Minor Illness Centre
Luton, Bedfordshire, England

www.minorillness.co.uk

For Ian, Amber, and Jenny

With thanks to Team Johnson and all of the
staff and patients from Kingfisher Practice,
past and present

ISBN-13: 978-1507693650

ISBN-10: 1507693656

Disclaimer

Every effort has been made to ensure that the information in this book is accurate. This does not reduce the need to exercise clinical judgment, and neither the author nor the National Minor Illness Centre accept any legal responsibility for any personal injury or damage arising from the use of the advice and information in this book. This advice relates only to the care of children in the United Kingdom.

Cover design by
Rochi Comunale and Kathryn Johnson

Cover image © istockphoto

CONTENTS

INTRODUCTION

In 2014 the UK Department of Health identified the management of minor illness as one of the six "Early Years High Impact Areas" for health visitors.

"Health visitors are a trusted source of knowledge, advice and information for parents and are often the first point of contact for parents who are unsure on the best course of action when their child is unwell. As such they play an important role in the primary care team and can help to reduce the burden on busy GP surgeries and A&E departments."

This book was written in response to the need for reliable, accessible information for health visitors when they are advising the parents of children with minor illness.

The information contained here is evidence-based, concise and targeted to guide the sometimes difficult decisions which health professionals often need to make about the assessment, home care, prescription or referral of an unwell child. Please visit minorillness.co.uk/health-visitors for our e-learning course, images of skin conditions, and references.

MINOR ILLNESS FUNDAMENTALS

A minor illness is a self-limiting condition which does not require intervention and can safely be managed at home. The most important skill is to distinguish it from more serious conditions.

In order to manage minor illness, you will need to be able to:

- Recognise the need for intervention because of:
  - Sepsis
  - Dehydration
  - A need for a test
  - A need for medication which you are unable to prescribe
- Provide evidence-based advice
- Prescribe appropriately
- Signpost to the most appropriate referral pathway

Using only your:
- Common sense
- Intuition
- Eyes
- Ears
- Hands
- Thermometer
- Torch

As well as doing basic nursing observations, you will need some specific examination skills:

- To examine the throat, to identify inflammation and purulence
- To assess for dehydration
- To check capillary refill time
- To identify chest recession

See the *Spotting the Sick Child* website to learn these techniques: www.spottingthesickchild.com

Normal values in under fives

Age (years)	Maximum respiratory rate	Maximum pulse
Under 1	40	160
1-2	35	150
2-5	30	140

Capillary refill time: normally less than 2 seconds. If it is prolonged on the hand, check again on the chest or forehead.

Temperature: normally below 37.5°C in the axilla.

FEVERISH ILLNESS IN CHILDREN UNDER FIVE

NICE CG160 (2013)

To ensure safe practice you must first familiarize yourself with this important document and the "traffic lights" assessment– see the back page of this book.

MEASURING TEMPERATURE

- Always use an axillary, not tympanic, thermometer in babies under four weeks (NICE, 2013)
- Use an axillary or tympanic thermometer in older children (RCN, 2013)
- Do not use mercury thermometers, oral or rectal thermometers or head strips (RCN, 2013)
- Axillary temperature is about 0.3°C below tympanic temperature

FEVER

- Fever in response to infection is part of the body's immune response and is **not**, in itself, dangerous
- The height of the fever does **not** predict serious illness, **except** in babies under six months (NICE CG160, 2013)
- Fever benefits the immune response, and there is some evidence that giving antipyretics may delay recovery (NICE CG160), 2013)
- There is **no** evidence that giving antipyretic drugs will prevent febrile convulsions (NICE CG160, 2013)
- Febrile convulsions do not cause long-term neurological problems

- **BUT** babies aged under six months are difficult to assess, and so, in them, fever should prompt urgent medical assessment
- This is not because the temperature itself is dangerous, but because it may indicate serious infection
- Clinical assessment is more difficult in young babies, so hospital tests may be needed

---

FEVER IN BABIES

Temperature greater than or equal to 38°C under age 3 months = red light

OR

Temperature greater than or equal to 39°C under age 6 months = amber light

This applies even after vaccinations – it is **not** safe to assume that a fever is related to the vaccine.

ANTIPYRETIC MEDICINES

- Routine lowering of fever is **not** recommended (NICE, 2013)
- Do not use tepid sponging (NICE, 2013)
- Paracetamol or ibuprofen may be given, but are **only** recommended to relieve pain or distress, not fever (NICE, 2013)
- Lack of response to antipyretic medicines does not predict serious illness (NICE, 2013)
- Giving ibuprofen and paracetamol simultaneously is **not** recommended (NICE, 2013)
- Only consider alternating these agents if the distress persists or recurs before the next dose is due (Wong, 2013)
- Prophylactic administration of antipyretics around the time of vaccination is no longer thought to lower antibody responses (Prymula, 2014), and new DH guidance recommends paracetamol cover for the first two Meningitis B vaccinations
- Paracetamol and ibuprofen packs often tell parents not to use them for more than two days without seeing a doctor. This advice is over-cautious and designed to avoid missing serious illness. If, by your assessment, the child does not have any "traffic light" symptoms, these products may safely be used for longer than this.

Paracetamol (first choice)

- Use in the first year of life is associated with an increased incidence of asthma, although causation has not been proved (Gonzalez-Barcala, 2012)
- The dosage regime was changed in 2011. Check with BNFC or NPF
- **Check what dose parents have been giving.** Children are often underdosed
- If indicated, encourage parents to buy it over the counter (OTC) for about £2 (UK prices)
- Known as acetaminophen in the USA

Ibuprofen

- Gives relief from pain and distress for about six hours
- Contraindicated if:
    - Chickenpox
    - Shingles
    - Gastroenteritis
    - Within 48hr of injury or operation
- Caution in asthma (rarely exacerbates wheeze)
- Many more cautions and contraindications apply to adults. See BNF or NPF
- If indicated, parents can buy OTC (£2)

For more information on OTC medicines, see www.medicinechestonline.co.uk

HOME CARE OF THE FEVERISH CHILD

- Look for signs of dehydration
- Offer regular fluids, and encourage a higher intake if signs of dehydration develop
- Dress the child appropriately to prevent overheating or shivering
- Avoid using fans or tepid sponging
- **Fever is not dangerous ("the immune system is busy") and does not need to be treated**
- Consider giving paracetamol (OTC, £2) or ibuprofen (OTC, £2) in full dosage if the child is in pain or distressed
- Do not use paracetamol and ibuprofen simultaneously
- Only consider alternating them if the distress persists or recurs before the next dose is due. Write the times of the doses down to avoid overdosing
- Check the child regularly, including during the night
- Keep the child away from day care while fever persists, and notify the nursery or childminder of the illness

Give worsening advice to the parent, as appropriate to the illness. Ensure that they have details of the opening hours and phone numbers for your local referral centres.

ASSESSMENT OF THE FEVERISH CHILD

NICE CG160 is the most important document for the identification of serious illness in the under fives. See the "traffic light" chart on the back page of this book.

CG160 states that the routine assessment of a child with a fever should include:

- Temperature
- Heart rate
- Respiratory rate
- Capillary refill time

The areas of assessment are:

- Colour
- Activity
- Respiratory
- Hydration
- Other

NICE "TRAFFIC LIGHT" ASSESSMENT

- **Red light** + an immediately life-threatening illness:
  dial 999

- **Red light** + no immediately life-threatening illness:
  take to A&E or refer immediately by phone to GP

- **Amber light:**
  see specialist nurse or GP within a few hours (e.g. GP surgery, Urgent Care Centre, Walk-in Centre)

- **Green light:**
  reassure, give worsening advice

REFERRALS

Keep a list in your diary of the local urgent care organisations, their opening times and contact phone numbers.

WHEN TO REFER THE FEVERISH CHILD

- NICE traffic lights amber or red

- Temp ≥ 38°C under 3 months

- Temp ≥ 39°C under 6 months

- Temp ≥ 40°C in an older child

- Fever for over 24 hours without obvious cause

- Fever for over 5 days (consider UTI)

- Travel to a malarial or tropical area in the last 12 months, plus no obvious cause for fever

MENINGOCOCCAL INFECTION

This is very rare in primary care, but is also the leading cause of death from infection in early childhood (NICE CG102, 2010). It carries a mortality of 10% and a 20% risk of long-term complications.

History:
- Fever, severe headache, vomiting, diarrhoea
- Refusing food and drink
- Limb pain (may be severe)
- Too ill to stand up
- Drowsiness, photophobia (late signs)
- In babies:
  - Irritability
  - High-pitched cry

Examination:
- NICE traffic lights
- Check carefully for a non-blanching rash. If dark skin, check the palms, soles and conjunctivae
- Rash is not always present, and in the early stages it may not be typical (i.e. it may blanch and may not be purple)
- Extremities may be cold and mottled
- In babies, fontanelle may bulge

Refer: urgently if suspected

SEPSIS

Sepsis in small children may occur from a wide range of illnesses (such as pneumonia, urinary tract infection, or meningitis). Many different micro-organisms may cause meningitis, not just meningococcus.

The signs of sepsis, whatever the cause, will be detected by using the NICE traffic lights assessment.

IMMUNOSUPPRESSED

It is very important to identify the immunosuppressed children, as their minor illness may rapidly become serious.
There are two types of immunosuppression:

- Due to medical conditions which reduce the immune response, e.g. prematurity, malnutrition, HIV, 22q syndrome, spleen problems, agammaglobulinaemia, SCID, leukaemia

- Due to medication: e.g. taking long-term prednisolone, during chemotherapy and for six months afterwards

RESPIRATORY AND EAR NOSE AND THROAT PROBLEMS

SORE THROAT

This is a very common condition which is usually viral, especially in under 5s, and lasts 5-10 days.

History
- Fever
- Cough or cold
- Is the child immunosuppressed?
- Do they have a heart valve problem?
- Is there a rash? (scarlet fever?, page 27)

Examination
- NICE traffic lights
- Do **not** examine throat if sick/drooling
- Red, inflamed throat?
- Purulence (white spots on tonsils)?

Home care
- Avoid food or drink that is too hot
- Eat soft food
- Offer honey (but not if aged under one year) (Food Standards Agency, 2010)
- Ice lollies or ice cream for older children
- Avoid smoky environments
- Five out of ten children will have recovered after four days

Prescription/OTC:
- Paracetamol or ibuprofen (both £2 OTC) for pain relief

ANTIBIOTIC FOR SORE THROAT

Most sore throats are caused by viruses, and an antibiotic will provide no benefit to these children.

- Pros:
    - An antibiotic may reduce the illness duration, but by less than one day
- Cons:
    - Only one child in 14 will benefit from an antibiotic
    - They may cause side effects and allergic reactions
    - Parents should also consider the hassle of getting an appointment and waiting to be seen, waiting to collect a prescription, and persuading their child to take a ten day course of medicine
    - Over-use of antibiotics increases the spread of resistance
    - The child's own "friendly bacteria" in the gut are likely to become resistant, which may cause a problem if they later develop a serious illness

FEVER/PAIN SCORE FOR SORE THROAT

This score is derived from a combination of the child's symptoms and your findings on examination:

- **F**ever during previous 24 hours
- **P**urulence (white spots on tonsils)
- **A**ttends rapidly (within three days)
- **I**nflamed tonsils
- **N**o cough/cold symptoms

One point is given for each positive answer.

Action:

If score ≥4 points, refer for antibiotics (60% are bacterial)

If score 2 or 3, consider referral for antibiotics if not improving in 1-2 days (40% are bacterial)

If score 0 or 1, not likely to benefit from antibiotics (<20% are bacterial)

(Little, 2013)

SORE THROAT – REFERRAL

Refer:

- Urgently to A&E if:
  - Child is very sick, drooling and unable to swallow saliva (epiglottitis? Do not examine the throat!)
  - NICE traffic lights amber or red
  - Breathing difficulty

- Within 24hr if:
  - Immunosuppressed
  - Heart valve disease
  - Scarlet fever rash (see page 27)
  - Fever/PAIN score 4 or more

- In 1-2 days if:
  - Fever/PAIN score 2 or more and not improving

Do not refer: just because of white spots on the tonsils

Scarlet fever

A bacterial infection (group A streptococcus), which is mainly seen in children aged 2-8 years.

History
- Sore throat, enlarged neck nodes
- Fever, headache
- Then rash starting on abdomen and chest, peels after 7 days

Examination:
- NICE traffic lights
- Rash: blanching rough red pinpricks
- Flushed face, pale around the mouth, "strawberry tongue"
- Red throat, maybe with macules over the hard and soft palate

Home care:
- Exclude from day care for 24hr after treatment
- Should resolve after about seven days

Refer: always, if suspected, for antibiotic. Notifiable disease (though not in Scotland)

Swollen Neck Glands

Enlarged lymph nodes in the neck indicate that the immune system is responding to an infection, often a sore throat. They commonly accompany viral infections, and may fluctuate in size as new infections are encountered.

Refer if:
- NICE traffic lights amber or red
- One single node is hard and enlarging
- Persistent enlargement for more than three weeks

This is a viral infection which causes painful swelling of the parotid salivary glands. It is most infectious from 2 days before symptoms develop until 9 days after.

History:
- Dry mouth, worse on swallowing or chewing
- Fever
- Malaise and headache
- Facial swelling
- Maybe abdominal or testicular pain

Examination:
- NICE traffic lights
- Tender swelling in front of the ear, may be asymmetrical

Home care:
- Maintain fluid intake
- Avoid acidic fruit juices
- Stay away from day care for five days after the onset of swelling

Prescription/OTC:
- Give paracetamol or ibuprofen (both OTC, £2) for pain relief

Refer if: suspected. Notifiable disease

OTITIS MEDIA

A common viral or bacterial infection of the inner ear.

History:
- Pain deep inside ear – often screaming
- Pulling, tugging, or rubbing of the ear (but this may be due to teething)
- Has the child been feverish or restless?
- Any vomiting? Are they off their food?
- Has there been a sudden discharge and/or loss of hearing in one ear?
- Is the child immunosuppressed?

Examination:
- NICE traffic lights
- Check behind the ear for mastoid swelling and tenderness

Home care:
- Children with active otitis media should not fly
- Children with discharge should not swim for at least two weeks
- 7 out of 10 children will have recovered after four days

Prescription/OTC:
- Give paracetamol or ibuprofen (OTC, £2) regularly in full dosage for pain

Refer:
Urgently if:
- NICE traffic lights amber or red
- Immunosuppressed
- Mastoid tenderness or swelling

Within 24hr if:
- Severe vomiting
- Persistent symptoms >4 days (30% of children)
- Aged under two years
- Discharge from the ear
- Hearing loss

Antibiotics in otitis media

Most otitis media is caused by viruses, and antibiotics are of minimal benefit.

- 60% of all children with otitis media will be free of pain within 24 hours (this figure is not improved by taking antibiotics)
- Only one child in 15 will benefit from antibiotics, and one or two out of 15 who take them will get side-effects
- Antibiotics do not reduce the risk of long-term complications
- Antibiotics are associated with a 50% increased risk of recurrence over 3 years (although it is not known if this is causal)

COMMON COLD

Healthy children may have 8 or more colds per year. 3 out of 10 will be better in four days and 7 out of 10 in a week.

History:
- Sneezing and blocked nose
- Sore throat
- Cough
- Watering eyes
- Maybe fever and muscle pain
- Babies may have difficulty in taking feeds

Examination: NICE traffic lights

Home care:
- Give paracetamol or ibuprofen (both OTC, £2) if needed for pain relief
- Consider sodium chloride nose drops for babies before feeds (OTC, £3)
- Consider nose clearing device
- Consider using Vicks VapoRub® (OTC, £3) in children aged 2 and above (Paul, 2010)
- Snufflebabe® has a different formula, and evidence is lacking
- Care with Olbas® oil, Karvol® etc. – can cause serious problems if put into eyes and nose

Do not refer: just because of green nasal discharge

History:
- Onset and duration
- Fever
- Sore throat and cold symptoms
- Headache
- Joint and muscle pains
- Is the child immunosuppressed?
- Specific questions:
  - Rigors
  - Foreign travel (see below)
  - Urinary symptoms

Examination: NICE traffic lights

Home care:
- Advice as for colds
- Maintain adequate fluid intake

Refer if:
- NICE traffic lights amber or red
- Immunosuppressed
- Rigors
- Travel to malarial or tropical area in previous 12 months
- Urinary symptoms

In 'flu pandemics, check the Public Health England website for current advice.

Cough

History:
- Duration
- Are they producing sputum? Colour?
- Vomiting after coughing
- Hoarse
- Chest pain
- Fever
- Breathlessness
- Is the child immunosuppressed?

Examination:
- NICE traffic lights
- Raised respiratory rate is a useful sign. Do you feel breathless watching them?
- Check for intercostal or subcostal recession

Home care:
- Keep out of smoky atmospheres
- Increase humidity e.g. run shower in bathroom (but don't use steam inhalations)
- Consider using Vicks VapoRub® (OTC, £3) in children aged 2 and above (Paul, 2010)
- Cough mixtures should not be given to children under six (MHRA 2009)
- Offer honey at night, if aged over one year

SPECIFIC TYPES OF COUGH

- Acute bronchitis
- Pneumonia
- Asthma exacerbation
- Croup
- Bronchiolitis
- Whooping cough

ACUTE BRONCHITIS

The commonest form of cough, caused by a viral or bacterial infection of the upper airways.

History:
- Fever
- Cough and maybe wheeze
- Maybe central chest pain on coughing
- Is the child immunosuppressed?
- Do they have sickle cell disease?

Examination:
- NICE traffic lights
- Check for intercostal or subcostal recession
- Respiratory rate, pulse and CRT should be normal

Prescription/OTC: none specific. Antibiotics are of no benefit

Refer if:
- NICE traffic lights amber or red
- Immunosuppressed
- Sickle cell disease (not trait)
- Bloodstained sputum
- Wheezy
- Persistent symptoms for >3 weeks

Do not refer because of green sputum, or a cough which persists for >1 week in a well child.

This is an infection of the substance of the lung, viral or bacterial, which has a high mortality. Pneumonia is 20 times more common than meningitis as a cause of serious infection in children under five (NICE CG47, 2007).

History:
- Fever
- Rigors
- Breathless
- Cough
- Maybe bloodstained or rusty sputum
- Unilateral chest pain

Examination:
- NICE traffic lights
- Look specifically for recession, raised pulse and rapid respiratory rate

Refer urgently: always if suspected, for chest examination, antibiotics and possible hospital referral

ASTHMA EXACERBATION

This is often caused by a viral infection and an antibiotic is rarely needed, but specialist assessment is required in order to judge the need for oral steroids and hospital referral.

History:
- Cough
- Wheeze
- Breathlessness
- Sleep disturbance
- Fever
- Previous hospital admissions for asthma

Examination:
- NICE traffic lights
- Look for recession, rapid respiratory rate, external wheeze
- Ability to complete a sentence

Home care:
- Salbutamol inhaler with spacer:
  - 2 puffs every 2 min, up to 10 puffs
  - Give puffs one at a time

Refer: for assessment and possibly oral prednisolone. Urgency of referral depends on your assessment

CROUP

A viral infection of children aged between 3 months and 5 years; mainly occurs in winter.

History:
- Cough (often 'brassy' or 'barking')
- High pitched crowing noise on inspiration, worse at night (stridor) .
- Maybe breathless
- Maybe mild fever

Examination:
- NICE traffic lights
- Look for recession, raised respiratory rate

Home care:
- Sit child upright
- Ample fluids
- Increase humidity, e.g. run shower in bathroom
- Steam inhalations are no longer recommended, because of poor evidence base and risk of scalds

Refer: if suspected, for oral steroids. Urgency of referral depends on your assessment

BRONCHIOLITIS

A viral infection of babies (mostly aged 3-6 months), mainly in winter. There is no effective treatment, but in severe cases hospital observation may be needed in case the child deteriorates and needs ventilatory support (NICE, 2015)

History:
- Starts with a cold for 2–3 days, then:
- Dry, wheezy cough
- Nasal discharge
- Possibly fever
- Breathlessness is often present, which may affect feeding

Examination:
- NICE traffic lights
- Usually a raised respiratory rate
- Look for recession

Home care:
- Sit child upright
- Ample fluids
- Steam inhalations are no longer recommended because of poor evidence base and risk of scalds

Refer: always, if suspected, to assess severity. Urgency of referral depends on your assessment

This is caused by a bacterial infection. Most confirmed cases are in adults, but there were 14 deaths in UK babies under 3 months in 2012 (CKS).

History:
- Thick sputum
- Coughing > 2 weeks, especially if whoop heard or vomiting occurs after coughing
- Even if fully immunised

Examination:
- NICE traffic lights
- Usually normal

Home care:
- Sit child upright
- Increase humidity e.g. run shower in bathroom
- Steam inhalations are no longer recommended because of poor evidence base and risk of scalds
- Ample fluids
- If <3/52 history, a minimum of 5 days day care exclusion is needed

Refer: if suspected. Notifiable disease. Antibiotic treatment reduces infectiousness, but does not hasten the child's recovery

Cough – Referral

Refer if:
- NICE traffic lights amber or red
- Immunosuppressed
- Sickle cell disease (not trait)
- Bloodstained sputum
- Any diagnosis other than acute bronchitis
- Persistent symptoms for more than three weeks

Do not refer just because of green sputum, or a cough which persists for over a week in a well child.

Parents may be surprised to find out how long coughs usually last. 30% of children with a cough will be better in one week, 70% in two weeks and 80% in three weeks.

ALLERGIC RHINITIS

Hay fever is unusual in children under seven, but other allergies (e.g. to pet fur) may cause similar symptoms.

History:
- Suspected trigger
- Timing
- Sneezing
- Red irritable eyes
- Itchy throat

Examination: check eyes for discharge (to exclude infection)

Home care:
- Avoid triggers if possible
- If pollen allergy suspected:
  - avoid walking in grassy, open spaces
  - keep windows shut when pollen count is high
  - change car pollen filters with each service
- Useful website: Itchysneezywheezy.co.uk

Prescription/OTC: oral antihistamine e.g. chlorphenamine (OTC, £4 from age one)

Refer: if diagnosis in doubt, or not responding

INFECTIVE CONJUNCTIVITIS

This is usually caused by a viral infection.

History:
- Sore eyes but no impairment of vision
- Discharge
- Maybe cold symptoms

Examination:
- Red conjunctivae
- Discharge in/around the eyes

Home care:
- Wipe eyes with cotton wool soaked in cooled boiled water
- Don't share flannels or towels
- Resolves spontaneously within 2 weeks
- Day care exclusion is unnecessary (Public Health England, 2010)

Refer:
- Babies under one month old with red eyes (not just sticky eyes)
- Those with severe symptoms, to consider topical antibiotics (10% risk of adverse reaction, small chance of benefit)
- A baby over 9 months with a persistently watering eye (may be a blocked tearduct)

Do not refer: just for green discharge

ABDOMINAL PROBLEMS

DIARRHOEA AND VOMITING

95% of cases are viral: bacterial and protozoal infections account for the rest.

History:
- Duration
- Severity, episodes in 24 hours
- Preceding constipation
- Fluid balance
- Blood
- Fever
- Recent foreign travel
- Contacts
- Are they immunosuppressed? Diabetes?
- Recent broad-spectrum antibiotics
- Recent hospital admission
- Farm visit
- Pet reptile at home (salmonella risk)?

Examination:
- NICE traffic lights
- Check specifically for dehydration

Home care:
- Expect recovery in 4 to 7 days
- Exclude child from day care until 48 hours after symptoms settle
- If cryptosporidia infection, avoid swimming in public pools for 2 weeks
- Worsening advice

- Extra fluids should be taken: 50ml/kg/4hr
- Avoid fruit juice and carbonated drinks
- Take small sips, not gulps
- Ice lollies may help if fluids not tolerated (may be made with rehydration solution)
- Fasting is no longer recommended – a normal diet should be resumed as soon as possible and babies should continue normal feeds
- Reassure about the gastro-colic reflex; parent may be alarmed that eating triggers an urgent need to pass a stool ("when she eats it just goes straight through her..."). This is harmless
- Hygiene:
    - In older children, encourage them not to turn on the tap with the hand they have just used to clean themselves
    - And to close the toilet lid before they flush! Particles may spray up to two metres away....
    - Consider using gloves to handle potties and dirty nappies
    - Take care when washing hands (both child and parent)
    - Use disinfectant or bleach in hot water every day to clean potties, toilet seats and handles, taps and toilet door handles
    - Soiled clothing should be washed separately at a minimum of 60°C

Prescription/OTC:
- Consider oral rehydration salts (OTC, £3 for 6 sachets) in:
    - Children under two, especially if under 6 months or underweight
    - Diarrhoea >5 times in 24 hours
    - Vomiting >2 times in 24 hours
- Do **not** use home-made solutions
- Probiotics have well-researched benefits (Allen and Martinez, 2010). There is no standard approved preparation – consider Actimel® /Yakult® from 6 months of age, but not if immunosuppressed.

Refer:
- Urgently if:
    - NICE traffic lights amber or red
    - Diabetes or immunosuppressed
    - Blood in stool (red or black) (suggests E. Coli infection, especially after a farm visit)
    - Green, red or brown vomit
    - Preceding constipation (overflow?)
- Within 24hr if:
    - Suspected food poisoning (notifiable disease, not in Scotland)
    - Recent travel outside Europe / North America /Australia / New Zealand
    - Recent broad spectrum antibiotics or hospital admission (*C. difficile?*)
    - Persistent symptoms >7 days

History:
- Stool frequency normally varies from 4/day in the first week to 2/day at age one
- Passing stools between 3/day and 3/week is normal by age four
- Two or more of the following indicate that the child is constipated:
    - Fewer than three stools per week (unless exclusively breastfed), typically type 2 or type 3 on the Bristol chart
    - Hard, large stools
    - 'Rabbit droppings' stools
    - Soiling

Examination: none

Home care:
- "Do not use diet alone as first-line treatment for constipation – changes in diet, lifestyle, and behavioural modifications should occur alongside the early use of laxatives" (NICE CG99, 2010)
- Treat promptly with a laxative, even if the history is very short
- Try increasing intake of fluids, and encourage drinking fruit juice containing sorbitol (e.g. prune, pear, or apple) in

children aged six months or above
- Recommend a high-fibre diet, but not bran
- Do not recommend changing milk formula, or cow's milk exclusion

Prescription:
- Compound Macrogol oral powder, half-strength is first-line
- But macrogols are not licensed in children under 2 years
- If ineffective, consider lactulose, docusate or senna
- Lactulose is licensed from one month of age, docusate from six months, and senna from two years

Follow-up:
- Follow-up is important – laxatives may be needed for several months
- Assess the toilet training regime, if appropriate
- Schedule toileting to train regular habits, e.g. after meals or before bedtime
- Suggest that parent keeps a bowel diary
- Suggest encouragement and reward systems, such as star charts, incorporated into toileting routines

Refer if:
- Problems from birth, or during the first few weeks of life
- Delay in passing meconium for more than 48 hours after birth in a full-term baby
- 'Ribbon' stools
- Abdominal distension with vomiting
- Suspected faecal impaction
- Suspected neuromuscular problem
- Not responding to your management

THREADWORMS

History:
- Perianal itching or discomfort, worse during the night
- Maybe more than one family member affected
- It is unusual to see worms in the perianal area during the day

Examination: none, but if the diagnosis is uncertain a tape test may be useful. Adhesive tape is applied to the perianal area first thing in the morning, and then examined under a microscope to detect threadworm eggs

Home care:
- No need to exclude from day care
- On the first day of treatment:
  - Wash all family's nightwear, bed linen, towels, and cuddly toys
  - Vacuum and dust thoroughly, especially the bedrooms; vacuum the mattresses
  - Thoroughly clean the bathroom by 'damp-dusting'; wash the cloth frequently in hot water
- Strict personal hygiene measures — for 2 weeks if combined with drug treatment or for 6 weeks if used alone:

- Wear a clean pair of close-fitting underpants or knickers every night
- Cotton gloves may help to prevent night-time scratching. Wash them daily
- Bath or shower immediately on waking each morning; wash around the anus to remove any eggs laid by the worms during the night
- General personal hygiene for all the family:
  - Wash hands and scrub under the nails first thing in the morning, after using the toilet or changing nappies, and before eating or preparing food
  - Discourage nail biting and finger sucking
  - Avoid sharing towels or flannels

Prescription / OTC: for children aged 6 months and under, hygiene measures alone are recommended (CKS). For older children, give a single dose of mebendazole (OTC, £6 for family pack from age two), repeated in 2 weeks if infestation persists. Treat all household members, even if asymptomatic

Refer: if aged 6 months to 2yrs (i.e. please contact GP to request a prescription); if a tape test is needed; or if not responding to treatment

COLIC

This distressing problem affects 10% of babies.

History / definition:
- Paroxysmal uncontrollable crying in an otherwise healthy infant aged under 3 months
- More than 3 hours of crying per day on more than 3 days per week for more than 3 weeks
- No association with feeding method (Drug and Therapeutics Bulletin, 2013)

Examination: none

Home care:
- Check for over-feeding
- For breast fed babies, try an exclusion diet for mother (dairy foods, eggs, nuts, wheat, soy and fish)
- There is no good evidence that Infacol®, lactase drops (Colief®), lactose free milk or acupuncture have any more than a placebo effect – but this effect may still be useful
- The same applies to cranial osteopathy (Dobson, Lucassen et al, 2012; Miller, 2014)
- Support the parents through personal visits and self-help groups e.g. Cry-Sis

Refer if:

- Weight <4th centile (or decreasing on centile charts)
- Head circumference >95th centile (or increasing on centile charts)
- Green or projectile vomiting
- Blood in stools
- Suspected cows' milk protein allergy:
  - Family history of asthma/eczema/hay fever
  - Urticaria
  - Eczema
  - Diarrhoea or constipation

REFLUX

This is a normal process which causes symptoms in over 40% of babies. It usually starts before 8 weeks and resolves by the age of one.

History:
- Regurgitation and vomiting
- Coughing and crying during feeds
- Poor feeding

Examination:
- Check weight on centile chart

Home care:
- Breastfeeding assessment, if applicable
- If formula fed, check quantities not excessive
- Try smaller, more frequent feeds
- If persistent, try thickened formula

Refer if:
- Severe or persistently projectile vomiting
- Red or green vomit
- Faltering growth
- Not improving, for Infant Gaviscon® trial
- Acid suppressants (e.g. ranitidine) are rarely needed. Only recommended for feeding difficulties (e.g. refusing feeds, gagging or choking), distress or faltering growth (NICE CG184, 2014)

URINARY TRACT INFECTION (UTI)

Urinary tract infection is of two types:

- Upper UTI: fever, loin pain, malaise
- Lower UTI: dysuria, urgency and frequency but no fever

Lower UTI (cystitis) is much more common than upper UTI (pyelonephritis). Although not often encountered, pyelonephritis is ten times more common than meningitis as a cause of serious sepsis in children under five (NICE CG54, 2009).

Pyelonephritis in children under 7 years may cause permanent kidney damage, which may lead to hypertension and renal failure. The younger the child, the greater the danger of scarring, and the more difficult it is to make the diagnosis.

Lower UTI symptoms, such as dysuria and frequency, are less common in small children and harder to detect.

UTI is commoner in children who have been sexually abused, but does not (in itself) raise safeguarding concerns unless there are other issues.

History:
- Dysuria
- Suprapubic pain
- Urgency
- Frequency of micturition
- Cloudy, red-brown or offensive urine
- Enuresis or wetting
- Fever and rigors
- Abdominal pain
- Vomiting
- Malaise
- In babies, maybe just:
  - Irritability
  - Poor feeding

Examination:
- If fever or suspected pyelonephritis, check NICE traffic lights
- Otherwise none

Home care:
- Adequate, but not extra, fluid intake
- Obtain a urine sample in a sterile bottle, ideally a clean catch sample. Washed-up potties are acceptable, but not if bleach has been used. Consider covering a potty or jug with clingfilm to collect the sample

Refer: always, if suspected, for urine testing and consideration of an antibiotic. Urgency of referral depends on your assessment

SKIN PROBLEMS

SKIN PROBLEMS - INTRODUCTION

It is crucial to take a good history **before** you look at the rash.

History:
- Parent's agenda (meningitis? contagious?)
- Duration
- Distribution
- Is the rash symmetrical (see page 69)
- Is the child unwell or feverish? If so, ask about recent travel to tropical area
- Is the rash itchy or painful?
- Are the spots of different ages?
- Have there been previous episodes?
- Are other family members affected?

Examination:
- If feverish or unwell, NICE traffic lights
- Distribution and symmetry
- Size
- Colour – if purple, are there tiny petechiae or larger areas (purpura)?
- Raised (papule) or flat (macule)?
- Can vesicles (blisters) be seen?
- Is surface scale present?
- Does the rash blanch on pressure?

Beware: it is very easy to underestimate the severity of a rash in a child with dark skin, because inflammation is much less obvious.

RASH IN AN UNWELL CHILD

Rashes are common in viral infections.

Some are typical:
- Slapped cheek
- Chickenpox
- Hand foot and mouth

Others are non-specific, and impossible to diagnose with certainty. Fortunately, in the UK in the 21st century, the vast majority of rashes do not signify serious infection. But *urgently refer* an unwell child with rash who has returned from West Africa in the last 3 weeks (?Ebola).

Common infectious causes:
- Slapped cheek (facial rash)
- Roseola infantum (baby recovering from feverish illness)
- Rubella (pink rash, swollen glands)
- Measles (high fever)
- Chickenpox (crops of itchy papules)
- Scarlet fever (sore throat and "sandpaper" rash, see page 27)
- Hand foot and mouth (characteristic vesicles, see page 91)

Very rare infectious cause:
- Meningococcal infection (a purpuric or petechial rash which does not blanch on pressure in a very sick child, see page 20)

SLAPPED CHEEK

A common rash caused by a parvovirus, most often in 4-10 year olds. The incubation period is 4-20 days. Once the rash has developed, the child is no longer infectious.

History:
- Runny nose
- Diarrhoea
- Headache
- Maybe fever, joint pains
- Then red rash on both cheeks

Examination:
- Bright red cheeks
- Later maybe a lacy rash on trunk and limbs

Home care:
- No specific treatment
- No need to exclude from day care

Refer if:
- Immunosuppressed
- Blood disorder
- Bone marrow problem

Also refer: pregnant contacts (less than 20 weeks – risk of miscarriage)

ROSEOLA INFANTUM

A common herpes virus infection in children aged three months to four years. The incubation period is around 12 days.

History:
- Sore throat
- Loss of appetite
- Enlarged neck glands
- Then sudden high fever which lasts 3-4 days

Examination:
- Rash usually appears when the fever subsides and the child is recovering
- Small pink macules appear on the body and spread to the limbs, not often on the face
- The rash usually only lasts for about 12 hours

Home care:
- No specific treatment
- No need to exclude from day care once rash has appeared

Refer if:
- Immunosuppressed
- Blood disorder
- Bone marrow problem

MEASLES

This causes the most severe illness of the UK rash-producing viruses, and is unlikely if the child has been immunised. The incubation period is 10 days; the child is infectious from several days before to four days after the rash appears. There were 1,843 confirmed cases in England and Wales in 2013, and one death.

History:
- Fever
- Malaise
- Loss of appetite
- Cough
- Runny nose
- Conjunctivitis
- Rash appears 1-4 days later

Examination:
- NICE traffic lights
- Koplik's spots may appear before the rash; blue-grey specks on a red base on the lining of the mouth
- Bright red maculopapular rash, first on the face then down the body, reaching palms and soles
- It peels off or fades after about a week

Refer if: suspected. Notifiable disease

RUBELLA

This viral infection is now uncommon in the UK. The child is infectious from 1 week before symptoms appear until 4 days after the onset of the rash.

History:
- Low-grade fever
- Headache
- Sore throat
- Runny nose and conjunctivitis
- Sometimes joint pains
- Any contacts who may be pregnant?

Examination:
- Rash starts behind the ears, before spreading to the face and neck and then to the rest of the body. It is pink and may be slightly raised, lasting 3–5 days
- Swollen lymph nodes may appear before the rash, and may last for 3 weeks or more. The nodes at the back of the skull, behind the ears, and in the neck are most often affected

Home care: no specific treatment

Refer if: suspected. Notifiable disease

Also refer: pregnant contacts (under 20 weeks)

CHICKENPOX

This infection is caused by the herpes zoster virus, with a long incubation period of 10-21 days. The child is infectious from 48 hours before the spots appear until 5 days after.

History:
- Malaise
- Fever
- Small red macules appear in crops
- These progress rapidly to papules, very itchy vesicles and pustules
- Rash crusts over after a few days
- Is the child immunosuppressed?
- Any contacts who may be pregnant?

Examination:
- NICE traffic lights
- Crops of papules and vesicles
- Check for superficial localised infection

Home care:
- Lukewarm baths may be soothing
- Try putting porridge oats in tights and holding under running bath water
- Exclude from day care for 5 days
- Contact with chickenpox will not cause shingles

Prescription/OTC:
- Avoid ibuprofen (increased infection risk)
- Chlorphenamine (OTC, £4, from age 1) or crotamiton (POM) may improve sleep and reduce the itch

- Virasoothe® (OTC, £8) is a new cooling gel on which no research has yet been published

Refer if:
- NICE traffic lights amber or red
- Immunosuppressed
- Breathless
- Confused
- Abnormal bleeding
- Secondary infection suspected

Also refer at-risk contacts, to consider zoster immunoglobulin.

5 minutes face-to-face or 15 minutes in the same room is regarded as significant exposure:

- Babies under four weeks (30% mortality if they develop chickenpox)
- Non-immune pregnant women (at any stage of pregnancy – high risk of complications for both mother and baby)
- Immunosuppressed

Purple Rashes

- Caused by blood escaping from the vessels, therefore the rash does not blanch when pressed (the "tumbler test")
- Petechiae (pinprick size) or purpura (larger areas)
- May be a sign of meningococcal septicaemia (child will be very ill); see page 20
- More commonly due to a low platelet count or auto-immune reaction
- Consider trauma / safeguarding issues, especially if the petechiae surround a bruise or if the distribution suggests attempted strangulation

Refer: urgently always, even if not unwell

- Purple rash + unwell/fever
  -> dial 999
- Purple rash + not unwell + no history of fever -> see a doctor within 2 hours (GP Update, 2015).

- Localised infections, asymmetrical distribution:
  - Shingles
  - Warts and verrucas
  - Molluscum
  - Impetigo
  - Fungal

- Itchy rashes, symmetrical distribution:
  - Infestations: scabies, head lice
  - Eczema
  - Urticaria

- Skin problems in babies:
  - Acne
  - Milia
  - Erythema toxicum
  - Umbilical granuloma
  - Cradle cap
  - Nappy rash

An asymmetrical distribution means that the pattern of the rash on the two sides of the body is not like a mirror image.

SHINGLES

A "re-awakening" of a previous chickenpox (herpes zoster) infection, which is common in older adults and unusual in children (though may even occur in babies).

History:
* Pain may precede the rash, which is confined to one dermatome
* May be mildly unwell
* Is the child immunosuppressed?

Examination:
* Unilateral
* Localised areas of blisters which gradually dry up and form scabs
* Limited area of inflammation around vesicles
* Exudate – straw coloured and translucent or purulent and opaque?

Home care:
* Infectious until the lesions have dried (usually 5–7 days)
* May cause chickenpox in others, but only by direct skin contact
* Avoid at-risk people (as for chickenpox, page 67)
* Avoid ibuprofen (increases infection risk)

- No need to routinely keep away from day care, unless the rash is weeping and cannot be covered, or if at-risk children or adults are attending (see page 67)

Refer if:
- Diagnosis uncertain
- Secondary infection suspected (inflammation spreading, purulent exudate)
- Severe rash or pain
- Immunosuppressed

WARTS AND VERRUCAS

Skin infections caused by human papillomavirus.

History: small, rough growths which usually develop slowly and may be painful

Examination: asymmetrical raised pale papules, or flattened areas on soles of feet or toes

Home care:
- Explain natural resolution, infectious nature
- Suggest that parent removes hard skin, e.g. with a Pedegg®, to increase comfort
- Consider using duct tape, or a square of banana skin taped on overnight with the white side against the skin
- No reason to exclude child from swimming – use a waterproof plaster

OTC:
- No treatment is best, but if causing discomfort:
- Salicylic acid paint, applied daily to affected area. This relieves pressure by dissolving hard skin, but does not cure the wart (Ashton and Leppard, 2014).

Refer if:
- Anogenital warts
- Immunosuppressed

A common localised viral infection.

History:
- Slowly-growing round lesions, usually on the trunk and in the flexures
- May be itchy

Examination:
- Asymmetrical
- Pearly white round raised lesions, may have central dimple
- Look for signs of secondary infection

Home care:
- Explain caused by a pox virus
- Infectious, so avoid sharing towels and flannels
- No need to exclude from day care
- Best left alone, will go in 18 months without scarring

Refer if:
- Immunosuppressed
- Signs of secondary infection
- Anogenital lesions (although not usually associated with abuse)

IMPETIGO

This is a bacterial infection of the skin, usually caused by staphylococcus or streptococcus, which most commonly occurs on the face. More serious bacterial infections may occur, secondary to a wound or a viral blister such as chickenpox.

History:
- Spreading sore area, which weeps then develops golden crusts
- The child may be unwell if a large area of skin is affected

Examination:
- Asymmetrical
- Well-defined, raw areas with crusting
- Maybe pustules (blisters full of purulent fluid)
- Check for cellulitis (a spreading area of redness and heat)

Home care:
- Remove crusts with soapy water
- Advice about cross-contamination; avoid sharing flannels and towels
- Exclude from day care until 48hr after the first treatment

Refer: always if suspected, for antibiotic (topical or oral)

FUNGAL INFECTION

History:
- Slowly spreading red or pink itchy patch which enlarges to become ring-shaped

Examination:
- Asymmetrical
- Often a clear central area and a scaly red edge

Prescription/OTC:
- Clotrimazole or miconazole cream (OTC, £4)
- Continue to treat for 2 weeks after apparent cure

Home care:
- Wash the affected area daily and dry thoroughly afterwards
- Wash clothes and bed linen frequently
- Avoid sharing flannels and towels
- No need to exclude from day care

Refer if:
- Diagnosis uncertain
- Not responding to initial treatment

SCABIES

This is caused by a mite which burrows under the skin, mainly on the fingers but maybe on the feet in babies. The mites may be present without causing symptoms for several weeks, before a generalised allergic reaction develops.

History:
- Intense itching, especially at night
- Other family members affected
- Very small babies may seem miserable and feed poorly
- Variable rash

Examination:
- Burrows may be seen on or between the fingers (maybe the feet in babies), or the flexor surfaces of other joints
- Spreading rash, often papular and usually scratched
- Widespread redness, particularly on the trunk
- Multiple crusted nodules on the trunk and limbs
- In babies, pink-brown papules and pustules may be seen, mainly on the palms and soles
- Look for signs of localized secondary infection

Home care:
- Hot wash for clothes and bedding
- Treat the whole family, even pregnant or breastfeeding mothers, and give a leaflet
- Exclude from day care until first treatment completed
- Warn about persistent itching, maybe for several weeks afterwards

Prescription / OTC
- Permethrin 5% (Lyclear Dermal Cream®) Apply to the whole body, including the scalp, face, neck, and ears. In small children, mittens may be needed to prevent them from sucking off the cream. Reapply after handwashing. Leave on for 12 hours, repeat after one week.
- Chlorphenamine (OTC, £4, from age 1) to reduce itching

Refer if:
- Treatment failure
- Secondary infection suspected

HEAD LICE

History:
- Itchy scalp
- Louse eggs, hatched (nits) or unhatched, although these alone are not sufficient to diagnose active infestation
- Live lice may be seen

Examination:
- Detection combing (systematic combing of wet or dry hair with a detection comb) will confirm the presence of lice
- The glands at the back of the neck may be enlarged

Home care:
- Best chance of success if all affected household members are treated on the same day
- Check whether treatment was successful by detection combing on day 2 or day 3 after completing the second treatment
- Check again after an interval of 7 days
- No need to exclude from day care once treated

Prescription/OTC:
- The child should only be treated if a live head louse is found
- All **affected** household members need simultaneous treatment
- All types of treatment need more than one session
- Dimeticone 4% lotion (Hedrin®, OTC, £9) Rub into dry hair and scalp, allow to dry naturally, shampoo off after at least 8 hours; repeat application after 7 days. Caution, flammable
- Or malathion 0.5% aqueous liquid (Derbac M®, OTC, £9)

Other possible OTC treatments:
- Wet combing using the Bug Buster® comb and method (OTC, £7)
- Full Marks® Solution (OTC, £7)
- Coconut, anise, and ylang ylang spray (Lyclear SprayAway®) (OTC, £15)

Do not recommend insecticidal shampoos or cream rinses, as they are less effective and may induce resistance.

Eczema

Atopic eczema is a chronic, relapsing, itchy skin condition. Children with atopic eczema have a reduction in the lipid barrier of the skin, which leads to excessive water loss.

History:
- Duration
- Itch
- Have any areas become painful?
- Previous treatments and effects

Examination:
- Distribution (usually symmetrical on the face and flexures)
- Severity
- Look for signs of infection (inflamed, weeping, crusted)

Home care:
- Avoid detergents and soaps. This includes bubble bath!
- Bathe or shower only two or three times per week
- Try putting porridge oats in tights and holding under running bath water
- Keep the child cool
- Praise them for not scratching. Consider a star chart

- Keep the fingernails short
- Choose cotton clothes rather than wool
- After swimming, rinse off any chlorine from the pool
- Useful website: Itchysneezywheezy.co.uk

Prescription/OTC:
Emollients are the first line treatment, applied at least three times a day, and stroked in the direction of the hairs.

Ointment, e.g. Zerobase® ointment, Diprobase® ointment (OTC, from £6), or Cetraben® cream (OTC, £9)
- If fire risk, use Oilatum® cream (OTC, £8)
- Large quantities of emollient, e.g. 250g per week, may be needed. Consider using "trial size" packs initially
- Pump dispensers are easier to use, and prevent contamination of the ointment
- If there is a sensitivity to one emollient, choose another with different additives
- Do not use preparations containing urea; they are much more expensive
- Preparations containing antiseptic should not be used unless the child gets recurrent infections
- Aqueous cream and ZeroAQS® are not recommended

Soap substitute, e.g. Hydromol Bath and Shower® (OTC, £6)
- The efficacy of bath additives is now questioned (Shams and Grindlay, 2011)

Refer:
- Urgently if:
  - Suspected bacterial infection (causes painful flare-ups)
  - Suspected eczema herpeticum (widespread vesicles in a sick child, due to herpes infection – **life-threatening**)
- If not responding to emollients (to consider topical steroids)

Topical steroids in eczema

- Secondary to emollient treatment
- Strong topical steroids (but not hydrocortisone) may cause skin atrophy or systemic effects
- Under-treatment may lead to scarring
- Eczema is a long-term condition. Parents often have unrealistic expectations of treatment
- Review is important, to arrange step-down or maintenance

URTICARIA (NETTLE RASH)

This itchy, transient rash is caused by histamine release from blood vessels in response to an allergic reaction.

History:
- Variable, itchy, raised rash of sudden onset
- New medicines?

Examination:
- Pale weals on red/pink flare
- Or maybe nothing to see

Home care:
- Try to identify triggers (heat, sun, pressure, food allergy)

OTC: antihistamine, e.g. chlorphenamine, (OTC, £4, from age one)

Refer: if the diagnosis is unclear or a prescription is needed

SKIN PROBLEMS IN BABIES

Acne

Newborn babies may develop acne when hair follicles get blocked with excess sebum and dead skin cells. This may be caused by the mother's hormones or a reaction to an oily cream. No treatment is needed.
Refer if: not clearing after 3 months

Milia

This affects half of all new babies. Pearly white cysts appear just under the surface of the skin, usually on the cheeks and eyelids. It is caused by the pores becoming blocked with keratin. No treatment is needed, and the milia disappear in a few weeks.

Erythema toxicum

This rash appears in babies 2-14 days old. Red blotches are seen, mainly affecting the face and body. Sometimes there are also papules, small pustules or vesicles, varying in size. The individual lesions can disappear within hours, and the baby remains well. No treatment is needed.

Umbilical granuloma

An umbilical granuloma is an overgrowth of tissue during the healing process of the umbilicus. It is most common in the first few weeks of life. It is a soft pink or red papule which is often moist and may leak small amounts of clear or yellow fluid. It has traditionally been treated with silver nitrate, but concerns about chemical burns have led to trials using home treatment with salt (Marzban, 2008).

Home care:
- Keep the belly button clean and dry
- Clean the area with soap and warm water when it gets soiled with urine or stool
- Expose to the air by rolling back the top of the nappy

If not improving, try salt treatment:
- Apply a small pinch of table or cooking salt
- Cover the area with a gauze swab and hold it in place for 10-30 minutes
- Clean the site using a clean gauze swab soaked in warm water
- Repeat the procedure twice a day for at least two days

Refer if: not responding

Cradle cap

This is a form of dermatitis which is caused by overactive skin glands.

History:
- Usually starts at 3-8 weeks of life
- Scaly rash on the scalp of a well baby
- Face, ears, neck, nappy area or flexures may also be affected
- Maybe mild itching

Examination:
- Yellow-brown, large greasy scales on scalp

Home care:
- Soften the scales with baby oil first, followed by gentle brushing, then wash off with baby shampoo
- If not improving, try soaking the crusts overnight with white petroleum jelly
- (Vaseline®, OTC, £2) and shampoo off in the morning
- May take several weeks to resolve

Prescribe/OTC: if previous treatments are ineffective

- Soap substitute, e.g. Hydromol Bath and Shower® (OTC, £6)
- Clotrimazole cream: apply twice daily (OTC, £3)

Refer if: symptoms persist longer than 4 weeks with treatment

Nappy rash

This is usually initially due to irritation from urine or diarrhoea, but after 48 hours it is commonly superinfected with candida (a type of yeast).

History:
- Check that the parent is not rubbing too hard on the skin or using rough paper, such as kitchen roll
- Itching?
- Distress?
- Consider nappy or cream allergy

Examination:
- Candidal superinfection is suggested by:
  - Distress
  - Pustules in the flexures
  - Satellite spots
- Bacterial superinfection is rare:
  - Marked inflammation
  - Vesicles and pustules may be seen
  - A bright red area may develop immediately around the anus

Home care:
- Leave the nappy off as much as possible and change frequently
- Avoid baby wipes – use cotton wool and water

- Avoid soap and bath additives, other than emollients
- Barrier creams should not be used routinely with disposable nappies.
- Sudocrem® contains an antiseptic and several potential skin sensitisers, including lanolin. Zinc and castor oil is preferred for mild nappy rash, but should not be applied thickly as this will reduce the absorbency of the nappy

Prescription/OTC:
- Soap substitute (e.g. Hydromol Bath and Shower®, OTC, £6)
- Titanium ointment (Metanium®, OTC, £3). Leave on as long as possible, then remove using baby oil
- If candida suspected, or not improving, use clotrimazole cream (OTC, £3) until at least two weeks after the rash has healed. Stop the barrier cream while using clotrimazole

Refer if:
- Suspected bacterial infection
- Red peri-anal area with itching and fissures (possible streptococcal infection, Lehman and Pinder, 2009)
- Not responding to treatment

Mouth Problems

Caused by candida, a type of yeast, and tends to be over-diagnosed.

History: baby with difficulty in feeding

Examination: white **adherent** patches on the tongue and lining of mouth

Home care: discuss dummy and teat sterilisation procedure, and if the mother is breastfeeding enquire about sore nipples (which would need separate treatment – do not suggest that she applies the oral gel to her nipples to treat the baby)

Prescribe/OTC, for at least 9 days:
- Miconazole oral gel (£4, OTC) (not licensed under 4 months). Smear inside the mouth 4 times daily, after food if possible
- Nystatin suspension (POM) is less effective. Although not licensed under one month, Community Prescribers are authorised to prescribe it in this age group (see NPF). Drop 1mL into mouth 4 times daily, after food if possible

Refer: if suspected and unable to prescribe

HAND, FOOT AND MOUTH DISEASE

A viral infection, usually caused by Coxsackie A16 virus, not related to foot and mouth disease in sheep.

History:
- Painful vesicles in or around the mouth then on the hands and feet
- Usually in a child who is mildly unwell

Examination:
- Crops of small vesicles on hands, feet, mouth and sometimes other areas

Home care:
- Symptomatic treatment
- Watch fluid intake if mouth is sore, and consider using cold drinks, syringe or straw
- No need to exclude from day care, unless contact with a woman in early pregnancy

Refer if:
- Immunosuppressed
- Blood disorder
- Bone marrow problem
- Secondary infection suspected

Also refer: pregnant contacts (in late pregnancy, baby may be infected)

PRIMARY HERPES SIMPLEX INFECTION

Most children will have been infected with the herpes simplex virus before the age of two. Often this causes no symptoms, but it may make them quite unwell. This is the primary infection which may lead to cold sores later in life.

History:
- Short history of fever
- Malaise
- Reluctant to eat or drink

Examination:
- Multiple small ulcers on tongue, palate, buccal mucosa
- Check for dehydration

Home care:
- Watch fluid intake – consider straw, syringe, or very cold drinks

Prescription/OTC:
- Paracetamol (OTC, £2) for pain relief

Refer if:
- Baby under four weeks
- Immunosuppressed

TEETHING

This frequently causes discomfort in infants aged 4 months to 3 years, but be careful to exclude other, more serious diagnoses.

History:
- Crying in pain
- Increased biting or sucking
- Drooling
- Rubbing gums
- Irritability
- Wakefulness
- Rubbing ears
- Red facial rash
- Off feeds
- Possibly a mild fever (but less than 38°C)

Examination:
- Temperature
- Check the mouth for signs of tooth eruption

Home care:
- Gentle rubbing of the gum with a clean finger
- Allow the baby to bite on a cool object, such as a chilled teething ring or a cold wet flannel
-
-

- In older babies, consider using chilled fruit or vegetables (e.g. banana or cucumber)

Prescription / OTC:
- Consider paracetamol (OTC, £2) or ibuprofen (OTC, £2) for pain relief
- Do not prescribe oral choline salicylate gel, because of the risk of Reye's syndrome
- Do not recommend topical anaesthetics (e.g. Bonjela®, Dentinox® or Calgel® teething gels)
- Severe adverse effects have been reported following inappropriate use of topical anaesthetics (CKS)

PRACTICALITIES

INFECTIOUSNESS

Exclusion from day care is usually "until better". A feverish child should not be in day care.

Specific exclusions are:

- Chickenpox - 5 days
- Hand foot and mouth disease - none
- Head lice – until after treatment
- Impetigo – 48hr after treatment
- Scabies – until after treatment
- Slapped cheek – none
- Whooping cough – 5 days if given antibiotics
- Diarrhoea/vomiting – until 48hr after resolution

Source: Public Health England (2010)

NOTIFIABLE DISEASES (UK)

- Food poisoning (even if only suspected, though not in Scotland)
- Measles
- Mumps
- Rubella
- Pertussis
- Scarlet fever (not in Scotland)
- Many other rare conditions

Nosebleed

Home care:
- Sit with the upper body tilted forward and mouth open. The child should avoid lying down, unless feeling faint
- Pinch the cartilaginous (soft) part of the nose firmly (not the bony part) and hold it for 10–15 minutes without releasing the pressure, breathing through the mouth

Refer to A&E if:
- Bleeding does not stop after 10 to 15 minutes of pressure
- Aged under 2 years (safeguarding concerns, (CKS))
- Profuse bleeding
- Bleeding disorder

Head injury

History:
- How and when did the head injury occur?
- From what height did they fall?
- Loss of consciousness
- Vomiting
- Headache
- Visual disturbance
- Bleeding disorder e.g. haemophilia

Examination:
- Normal level of consciousness
- Bruising around eyes or behind ears

Home care:
- Avoid contact sports, overexcitement and too much 'rough and tumble' play for the next few days
- Worsening advice – see NHS Choices, or give a leaflet
- Tell parent to attend A&E urgently if the child:
  - Becomes increasingly sleepy or confused
  - Complains of worsening headaches
  - Cries persistently
  - Vomits (more than twice)
  - Develops worrying symptoms, e.g. seizure, unsteady walking

Prescription/OTC: Paracetamol (OTC, £2) or ibuprofen (OTC, £2), if required for mild headache

Refer to A&E if:
- Safeguarding concerns (especially in a non-mobile child)
- Fall of more than one metre, or greater than the child's height
- Bleeding disorder
- Loss or impairment of consciousness
- Significant injury, bruise or swelling larger than 5cm
- Clear fluid running from the ear or nose
- Black eye or bruising behind the ear
- Bleeding from ear, or new deafness
- Visual disturbance
- Two or more episodes of vomiting since the injury
- Persistent headaches or irritability
- Any unusual worrying symptom

Burn

Home care:
- Irrigate the burn as soon as possible with cool or tepid water, by immersing the area if possible, for between 10 and 30 minutes. Do not use iced water
- Keep the child warm to avoid hypothermia if cooling large areas
- If dressing needed, cover the burn with cling film, but do not wrap it all round the limb
- Use a clean, clear plastic bag for hands
- If swollen, elevate the affected limb

Examination:
- Depth and extent of burn
- Are vesicles present?

Prescription/OTC: Paracetamol (OTC, £2) or ibuprofen (OTC, £2) for pain relief

Refer if:
- Safeguarding concerns
- Dressing needed
- Blisters / deep burn / burn goes completely around a limb
- Larger than two handprints (Hettiaratchy and Papini, 2004)
- Involving the face, hands, feet, perineum, genitalia, or any flexure
- Possible infection

Sunburn / heatstroke

History:
- Sun exposure
- Use of sunscreen
- Fluid intake

Examination:
- Temperature
- Pulse

Home care:
- Cool bath or shower
- Apply topical emollients and cold compresses
- Drink enough fluids

Prescription/OTC: Paracetamol (OTC, £2) or ibuprofen (OTC, £2) for pain relief

Refer if:
- Safeguarding concerns
- Suspected heatstroke:
  - Dizziness or fainting
  - Nausea or vomiting
  - Headache or muscle pain
  - Strange behaviour: irritability, confusion, hallucinations
  - High temperature
  - Rapid pulse

Prescribing or OTC?

Most of the medicines recommended in this book are available over the counter. If parents are prepared to buy the medicine, this will save the NHS a great deal of money. Busy parents may prefer to buy medicines rather than have to arrange an appointment, wait to be seen and wait again for a prescription to be dispensed.

However if you suspect that, unless you prescribe, the parent will book a GP appointment to obtain the medicine, then it would be much more cost-effective for you to prescribe. A prescription for paracetamol, for example, which costs only £2 over the counter, could cost the NHS £48 because of a GP consultation and a dispensing fee.

Approximate UK OTC costs are given in this book to aid you in advising the parents. They are, of course, subject to change. As a general rule medicines are cheaper in supermarkets than in pharmacies, although advice on the use of the medication will only be available if the supermarket has its own pharmacy. Whilst it is acceptable for you to answer queries on what services are available, it would be unprofessional to recommend any particular pharmacy.

PRESCRIBING NOTES

Abridged information is given here for convenience, but always check with the NPF.

Oral medicines for pain

Paracetamol oral suspension, 120mg/5mL; 100mL, 500mL. First choice. Not licensed under 2 months. Caution if underweight.

Paracetamol dosages

2-3 months	1.25 to 2.5mL	every 8 hours if needed	Max 3 doses in 24hr. Max daily dose 60mg/kg
3-6 months	2.5mL	every 4–6 hours if needed	max 4 doses in 24hr
6-24 months	5mL		
2-4 yrs	7.5mL		
4-5 yrs	10mL		

Ibuprofen oral suspension, 100mg/5mL; 100mL, 150mL, 500mL. Not licensed under 3 months, or weight under 5 kg. Max dose 30mg/kg/24hr. Cautions: allergy; clotting, kidney, heart, liver or stomach problems; active skin infection; within 48hr of injury or operation; asthma (rarely, exacerbates wheeze - ask if there has been a previous problem).

Ibuprofen dosages

3-6 months	2.5mL	3 times daily if needed
6-12 months	2.5mL	3-4 times daily if needed
1-4 yrs	5mL	3 times daily if needed
4-5 yrs	7.5mL	3 times daily if needed

Oral medicines for constipation

Compound Macrogol oral powder, half-strength; 30 sachets. First choice.
Not licensed under 2 years. Mix contents of each sachet in quarter of a glass of water.
  "Give 1 sachet daily; adjust dose to produce regular soft stools (max. 4 sachets daily)."

Lactulose solution, 3.1–3.7 g/5mL; 300mL, 500mL. May take up to 48hrs to act.
Child 1 month–1 yr: "*Give 2.5 mL twice daily, adjust according to response*""
Child 1–5 yrs: "*Give 2.5–10 mL twice daily, adjust according to response*"

Head lice

Dimeticone 4% lotion; 50mL, 120mL (spray), 150mL. Not licensed under 6 months. Avoid contact with eyes. Keep child's hair away from fire. "*Rub into dry hair and scalp, allow to dry naturally, shampoo off after 8 hrs. Repeat after 7 days.*"

Malathion 0.5% liquid; 50 mL, 200 mL.
"*Rub into dry hair, allow to dry naturally, wash off after 12 hr, repeat in 7 days*"

Scabies

Permethrin 5% cream; 30g.
Not licensed under 2 yrs. Avoid contact with eyes; do not use on broken or infected skin. If hands washed within 8 hours, re-treat.
Application should be extended to include scalp,

neck, face, and ears, despite the contrary information given in the pack leaflet.
"Apply over whole body, wash off after 8–12 hours. Repeat after 7 days."

Nappy rash

Zinc and castor oil ointment; 500g.
Caution – contains peanut extract.
"Spread thinly over sore area at each nappy change."

Titanium ointment BP; 30g. This is sticky - consider using baby oil to remove it.
"Spread thinly over sore area at each nappy change."

Emollients for eczema and dry skin

Zerobase® ointment; 50g, 500g (pump)
Cetraben® cream; 50g, 150g, 500g, 1.05kg (all sizes have pump packs)

If fire hazard:
Oilatum® cream; 50g, 150g, 500mL (pump), 1.05L (pump)

For all emollients: *"Stroke into skin at least three times daily, especially after a bath."*

Wash for eczema and dry skin

Hydromol® bath and shower emollient;
350mL, 500mL, 1L.
"'Apply to wet skin and rinse off."

Antifungal preparations

Clotrimazole 1% cream; 20g, 50g. For fungal infections and candida nappy rash. Avoid contact with eyes and mucous membranes.
"Apply three times daily. Continue for two weeks after healing."

Miconazole oral gel; 15g, 80g. For oral thrush. Not licensed under 4 months, or if baby was preterm, under 6 months. Not to be used on mother's nipples to treat the baby.
Child under 2 yrs: *"Smear 1.25mL inside the mouth 4 times daily, after food if possible, for at least 9 days or until 2 days after complete healing."*
Child 2-5 yrs: *"Smear 2.5mL inside the mouth 4 times daily, after food if possible, for at least 9 days or until 2 days after complete healing."*

Nystatin suspension, 100,000 units/mL; 30mL. For oral thrush.
"Drop 1mL into mouth 4 times daily, after food if possible, for at least 9 days or until 2 days after complete healing."

ABBREVIATIONS

BNF – British National Formulary
BNFC - British National Formulary for Children
CG – Clinical Guideline
CKS – NICE Clinical Knowledge Summaries (UK)
CRT – Capillary refill time
GP – General practitioner
HIV – Human immunodeficiency virus
NHS – National Health Service (UK)
NICE – National Institute for Health and Clinical Excellence (UK)
NPF – Nurse Prescriber's Formulary
OTC – Over the counter
POM – Prescription only medicine
SCID – Subacute combined immunodeficiency
UTI – Urinary tract infection

REFERENCES

Unless otherwise stated, the sources of reference are:

1.   Johnson G., Hill-Smith I. (Eds) (2012). *The Minor Illness Manual (4th edition).* Radcliffe Publishing Ltd, Oxford. ISBN-13: 978-1846195648

2.   **NICE CKS**: http://cks.nice.org.uk

Please visit minorillness.co.uk/health-visitors for other references, images of skin conditions, and our e-learning course.

INDEX

NICE CG160 TRAFFIC LIGHTS

Abbreviated Version	GREEN *low risk*	AMBER *intermediate risk*	RED *high risk*
Colour (of skin, lips or tongue)	• Normal colour	• Pallor reported by parent/carer	• Pale/mottled/ ashen/blue
Activity	• Responds normally to social cues • Content/smiles • Stays awake or awakens quickly • Strong normal cry/not crying	• Not responding normally to social cues • No smile • Wakes only with prolonged stimulation • Decreased activity	• No response to social cues • Appears ill to a healthcare professional • Does not wake, or if roused does not stay awake • Weak, high-pitched or continuous cry
Respiratory		• Nasal flaring • Respiratory rate >50/min, age 6–12 m >40/min, age >12 m • Oxygen saturation ≤95% in air • Crackles in the chest	• Grunting • Respiratory rate >60/min • Moderate or severe chest indrawing
Circulation and hydration	• Normal skin and eyes • Moist mucous membranes	• Tachycardia: >160/min, age <1yr >150/min, age 1-2yrs >140/min, age 2–5yrs • Capillary refill time ≥3 sec • Dry mucous membranes • Poor feeding in infants • Reduced urine output	• Reduced skin turgor
Other	• None of the amber or red symptoms or signs	• Age 3–6 m, temperature ≥39°C • Fever for ≥5 days • Rigors • Swelling of a limb or joint • Non-weight bearing limb/not using an extremity	• Age <3 m, temperature ≥38°C • Non-blanching rash • Bulging fontanelle • Neck stiffness • Status epilepticus • Focal neurological signs or seizures

16760370R00065

Printed in Great Britain
by Amazon